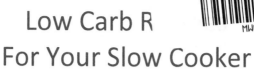

Low Carb R
For Your Slow Cooker

Tasty And Healthy Keto Meals
To Cook With Your Slow Cooker

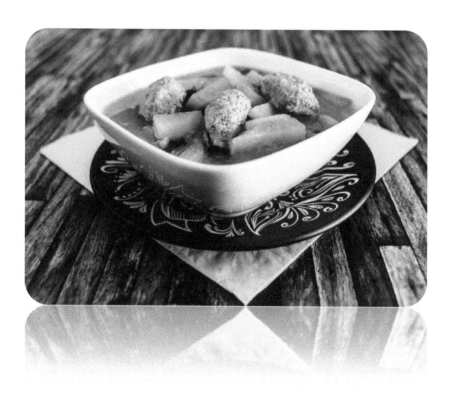

Main Dishes, Soups & Stews, Condiments & Sauces

Nana Ferretti

TABLE OF CONTENTS

The Slow Cooker

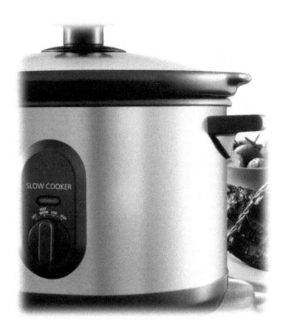

When it comes to dieting, some cooking methods are more suitable than others, e.g., grilling against frying. However, since Keto cooking is mostly about fats and then protein, you ideally want to try a convenient method that lets you preserve the nutritional goodness of your meals and, of course, the necessary fats. And this where slow cooking can come to the rescue. In particular, slow cooking has the following advantages when being on Keto, and you better try this out:

- It helps you control what goes inside and specifically the number of sugars and carbs. Since you will choose the ingredients to add, there will be no more guessing or having to read food labels to add low or zero sugar and carb ingredients like the ones listed earlier. This is perhaps the main advantage of using a slow cooker when on Keto. We have made this easier for you in this e-book by outlining the basic nutritional info for each recipe so you know exactly what goes inside.

- It maintains all the fats inside. By now, you have already realized that fats should be your main priority when on Keto. The issue with other cooking methods is that they dissolve and sometimes burn and evaporate the fat, e.g., grilling, which gets rids of the extra fat we need for keto and also makes the fat oxidize, which isn't healthy at all. On the contrary, slow cooking is one of the very few cooking methods that help preserve the original fat of the ingredients without oxidation, provided that you don't overcook your meals.

- It lets you prepare low carb yet fully nutritious liquids and sauces. A Slow Cooker can be used to make excellent chicken, beef, fish, and veggie stock, which are nutrient-dense yet contain little to none carbs—and yes, this is what we are looking for when on keto. You can later use any of these stocks as your base to cook healthy and delicious keto meats or veggie meals without adding carb-heavy sauces on top to add flavor. Since Slow Cookers work better with a bit of liquid, this kind of stocks and sauces can become your staples.

The Basics

Provided you use your slow cooker properly—and we'll attempt to outline all the basic steps as well as some tips and tricks, there is no reason why you shouldn't use your slow cooker when being on keto.

If you are new to slow cooking, you don't have to worry about any fancy cooking techniques as the slow cooker will work its magic on your own, and the steps of setting up are so easy, even a small kid can cook with it.

When you buy a slow cooker, most manufacturers feature a low or high setting to choose for cooking your food, besides the on/off button. This may vary a bit from brand to brand, but usually, this is the main setting of a slow cooker. Read the manufacturer's instructions first to make sure you use it properly.

In general, the low setting is applicable to foods and ingredients that don't need much time to be cooked properly in the oven. In most cases, the low setting should be between ½ to 3 hours max. These are:

- Fish and seafood

- Sausages

- Boneless and skinless or tender cuts of meat, e.g., tenderloin

- Thinly cut veggies

- Soup Mixes

On the other hand, high setting, which takes 3-8 hours in most cases, is suitable for chunkier and tougher veggie or meat pieces like:

- Beef cuts, e.g., steaks, cubes, briskets, prime rib, oxtails

- Pork Chops

- Whole pork shoulders or pork bellies

- Spare ribs

- Celery Stalks

- Carrots (sliced thickly)

As a rule of thumb, the tougher the cut is, the slower cook time it will need to get juicier and tender--the softer or smaller it is, the less cook time it will need after setting this on.

- For convenience reasons and if you are in a hurry, you can add all the ingredients that a recipe calls chopped (if using meats or veggies) or peeled and wholesome without any other preparation. However, there are some tips that will help you with the best results when it comes to flavor, texture, and cook time. Here are some:

- Brown your meats and/or veggie chunks first. This is optional, but this is actually what helps retain the flavor of meats and veggies and makes them taste more roasty instead of boiled. It may sound time-consuming, but it's not--it only takes a couple of minutes on high heat and a bit of oil to get them to change color.

- Use softer ingredients last or in large, thicker pieces. This will ensure that they don't become too mushy or fall apart after slow-cooking. Some green leafy veggies like spinach, which wilt easily, could also be added last (during the last 30 minutes to an hour).

- Fill ideally ⅔ of your slow cooker, so there is a little extra space for the food to cook freely. Filling it too much with solid and liquid ingredients will make the food steamed instead of simmered.

- Layer things properly. Some recipes are all about layering. In general, veggies (especially root vegetables) should come first, followed by meats and then liquids or spices.

- Don't raise the lid. You may be tempted to take a sneak peek or check if the food has been cooked properly, but if you do this more than once, you will end up losing valuable heat. Some recipes may require occasional stirring, but for most of the recipes, lifting the lid is unnecessary and a mistake.

- Use dairy in moderation. Some dairy products are fine when used in a slow cooker, while others will disintegrate and become a mess, so you better pay attention to the dairy products you add. Hard and fine cheeses like mozzarella and cheddar are fine when added last, but heavy creams and yogurts should be avoided altogether as they will break and fall apart.

- Use alcohol in moderation. While on a regular stovetop, alcohol will evaporate and add its aromas to the food without suffocating it; in a slow cooker using too much alcohol can make food taste just like that—pure, raw alcohol and cover the flavors and aromas of the rest of the dish. A little red or white wine is fine, but anything more than that should be avoided.

- Don't use poultry (chicken or duck) with the skin on unless you want to end up with a chewy, rubber-like skin that is also flavorless. If you want to add the skin, you can brown it first on a frying pan to make it crispier and flavorful.

- Don't overcook. Pay close attention to the recipe cook times and don't overcook something in hopes that it will get more tender and juicy—it will simply fall apart and become a mushy mess, especially if you are using fish or thinly cut veggies.

- Add the herbs last. Since herbs have a delicate flavor and aroma, putting them in the slow cooker too soon will dilute their scent to the point where you almost don't recognize it. Herbs, just like dairy, are best placed during the last 30 minutes of cooking.

- Last but not least, make sure you use some type of stock or any other liquid to submerge lean meat cuts, or your meat will dry up.

Benefits
of Using a Slow Cooker

Slow cooking is a cooking method invented in the 1970s and is still widely popular today for quite a few reasons. In general, slow cookers have the following benefits for you:

- Less cooking preparation. Since the slow cooker works mostly on its own, you don't have to spare a great deal of time to prepare the ingredients or stir them up or even sit and watch as the slow cooker will cook everything automatically in the hours you've set this. All you need to do is turn it on, dump in the ingredients, and set it to your desired setting while you are free to do other things, for example, doing house chores or babysitting the kids. This is, of course, handy for busy people who don't have the time and energy to prepare nice meals—and if your slow cooker automatically turns off after the time you have set it to cook, there will be no worries that your food will burn or fall apart.

- More succulent and juicier results. Slow cooking, as its name suggests, slow cooks the food for hours, and that helps it retain all its juices—dried up and chewy food will be a thing of the past when you are using a slow cooker. Slow cooker especially works its magic in tough cuts of meats that tend to get chewy when using other cooking methods like frying or baking, for example, pork chops, beef chuck, pork bellies, and bone-in chicken or poultry.

- More flavorsome results. The slow cooking process, apart from maintaining the juices and the soft texture of your meals, will also help preserve their flavor. And the best part is, you won't need a bunch of ingredients to prepare something delicious. The slow cooking process slowly releases and blends all the flavors and aromas you place inside, and everything literally melts together.

- A slow cooker can help save valuable energy. This may not be so obvious to some, but slow cookers have been found to consume less electricity than conventional ovens who "eat" more energy resources to function. This, of course, will help you save money on electricity bills in the long run, especially if you use your slow cooker in place of your regular oven at least once a week.

- Slow Cooker is generally safe. The issue with other cooking methods is that they can be dangerous when you don't pay attention, like frying and grilling, and kids should avoid using these without any supervision. A slow cooker, on the contrary, can be used by almost everyone, even kids, as it releases slow and gradual amounts of heat, and there are no spills or excessive heat that might cause burns (well, unless you touch it inside when it's on).

- It's easy to clean up—no need to wash it underwater and soap like the rest of your utensils. A simple cloth, liquid, water, and vinegar, or even baking soda are enough to wipe out any remaining fats and dirt.

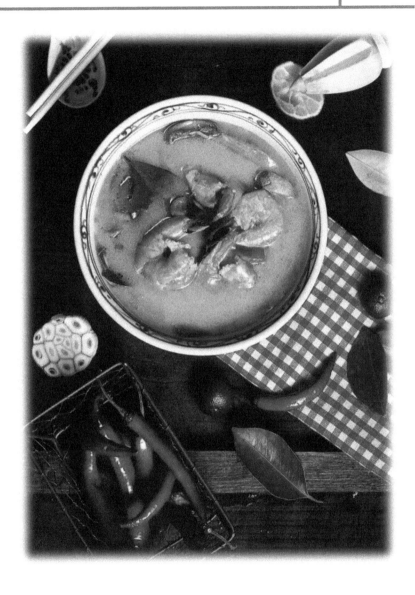

MAIN DISHES

Shrimp Bake

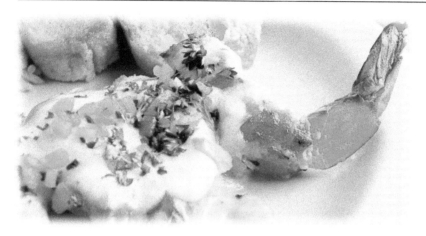

Prep time: 10 minutes

Cooking: 2 hours

Servings: 2

Ingredients:

- 1lb. shrimp
- 2 tbsp. lime juice
- 1 tsp. salt
- 1 tsp. apple cider vinegar
- 1 tbsp. butter
- ¾ cup heavy cream
- 2oz. provolone cheese

Directions:

1. Mix the shrimp with the lime juice and the other ingredients except the cheese.

2. Toss, sprinkle the cheese on top and cook on High for 2 hours.

Nutrients per serving:
- Calories: 290
- Fat: 5g
- Carbs: 3g
- Protein: 18g

Flavored Tilapia

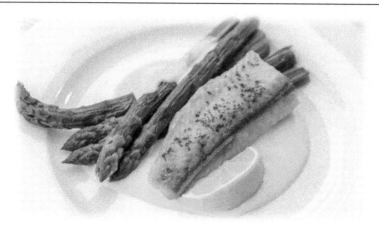

Prep time: 10 minutes

Cooking: 2 hours

Servings: 4

Ingredients:

- 1 asparagus bunch, spears trimmed
- 12 tbsp. lemon juice
- 4 tilapia fillets
- A pinch of lemon pepper
- 2 tbsp. olive oil

Directions:

1. Divide tilapia fillets on 4 parchment paper pieces.
2. Divide asparagus on top, drizzle the lemon juice, and sprinkle a pinch of pepper.

3. Drizzle the oil all over, wrap fish and asparagus, and place in your slow cooker.
4. Cover and cook on High for 2 hours.

Nutrients per serving:

- Calories: 200
- Fat: 3g
- Fiber: 1g
- Carbs: 8g
- Protein: 6g

Special Seafood Chowder

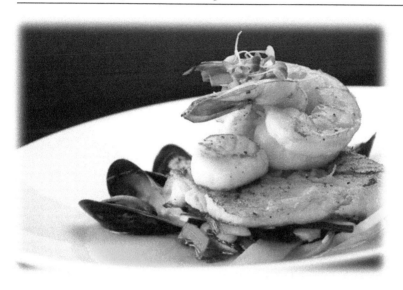

Prep time: 10 minutes

Cooking: 8 hours and 30 minutes

Servings: 4

Ingredients:

- 2 cups water
- ½ fennel bulb, chopped
- 1 yellow onion, chopped
- 2 bay leaves
- 1 tbsp. thyme, dried
- 1 celery rib, chopped
- Black pepper to the taste
- A pinch of cayenne pepper
- 1 bottle clam juice

- 2 tbsp. tapioca powder
- 1 cup coconut milk
- 1 lb. salmon fillets, cubed
- 5 sea scallops, halved
- 24 shrimp, peeled and deveined
- ¼ cup parsley, chopped

Directions:

1. In your slow cooker, mix water with fennel, onion, bay leaves, thyme, celery, clam juice, cayenne, black pepper, and tapioca powdered, stir, cover, and cook on Low for 8 hours.
2. Add salmon, coconut milk, scallops, shrimp, and parsley, cover, and cook on Low for 30 minutes more.

Nutrients per serving:

- Calories: 354
- Fat: 10g
- Fiber: 2g
- Carbs: 7.8g
- Protein: 12g

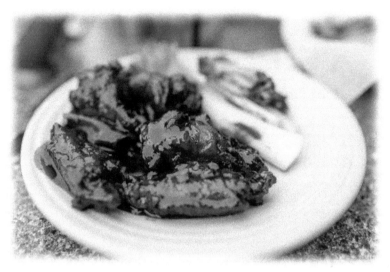

Chicken Casserole

Prep time: 5 minutes

Cooking: 3 hours

Servings: 3

Ingredients:

- 2 cubed boneless chicken breasts
- 1 can (8 oz.) tomato sauce
- Dash of pepper
- 1 tsp. Italian seasoning
- 1 bay leaf
- ¼ t. salt

For the garnish:

- ½ cup shredded mozzarella cheese

Directions:

1. Chop the chicken into cubes.
2. Pour in the sauce and spices. Stir and cook on the low setting for three hours.

Nutrients per serving:

- Calories: 228
- Fat: 8.8g
- Protein: 31.2g
- Carbs 6g

4-Ingredient Jerk Chicken

Prep time: 5 minutes

Cooking: 5 hours

Servings: 4

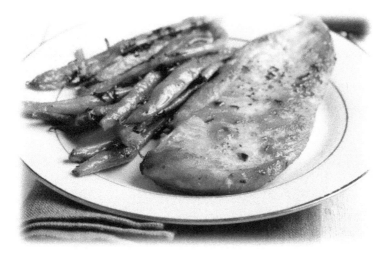

Ingredients:

- 5 chicken breasts
- 6 tsp. salt free Jerk seasoning spice
- 5 tsp. virgin olive oil
- 4 tsp. salt

Directions:

1. Rinse your chicken.
2. Mix with oil.
3. Rub Jerk seasoning and salt all over the chicken.
4. Cook on low for 5-6 hours.

Nutrients per serving:

- Calories: 200
- Fat: 12g
- Protein: 31g
- Carbs: 9g

Creamy Chicken Thighs

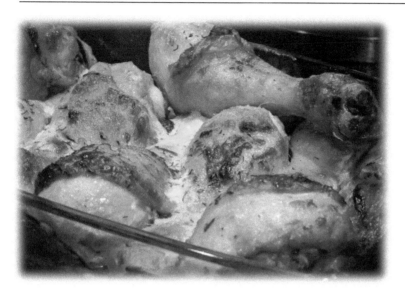

Prep time: 15 minutes

Cooking: 6 hours

Servings: 4

Ingredients:

- 1lb. chicken thighs, skinless
- ¼ cup almond milk, unsweetened
- 1 tbsp. full-fat cream cheese
- 1 tsp. salt
- 1 onion, diced
- 1 tsp. paprika

Directions:

1. Mix the almond milk and full-fat cream.

2. Add salt, diced onion, and paprika.

3. Stir well.

4. Place the chicken thighs in the slow cooker.

5. Add the almond milk mixture and stir it.

6. Cook the chicken thighs for 6 hours on High.

Nutrients per serving:

- Calories: 224
- Fat: 14.3g
- Carbs: 4.7g
- Protein: 18.9g

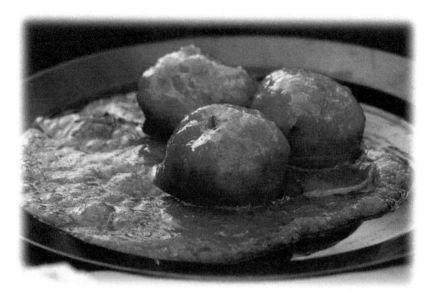

Meatballs Stuffed With Cheese

Prep time: 5 minutes

Cooking: 3 h on High/6 h on Low

Servings: 4

Ingredients:

- 2 1/2 lb. ground pork, pasture-raised
- 1/2 cup pork rinds, crushed
- 1/2 tsp. garlic powder
- 1/2 tsp. salt
- 1/2 tsp. ground black pepper
- 2 tbsp. Italian seasonings
- 2 cup marinara sauce, sugar-free and organic
- 2 eggs
- 1/2 cup grated Parmesan cheese

- 8 oz. block of mozzarella cheese, cut into 24 pieces

Directions:

1. Crack eggs in a large bowl, add pork rind, garlic powder, salt, black pepper, and Italian seasoning, and whisk until combined.
2. Add ground meat, then mix until combined and shape the mixture into 24 meatballs.
3. Place a piece of cheese into the center of each meatball and then wrap the meat around it.
4. Pour half of the marinara sauce into the bottom of a 6-quart slow cooker, then arrange meatballs and cover with remaining sauce.
5. Plug in the slow cooker, shut with lid, and cook meatballs for 6 hours at low heat setting or 3 hours at high heat setting.
6. Serve straight away.

Nutrients per serving:

- Calories: 548
- Fat: 12g
- Carbs: 6.5g
- Protein: 49g.

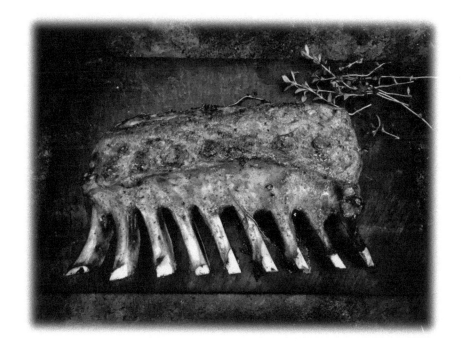

Spare Ribs

Prep time: 10 minutes

Cooking: 8 hours

Servings: 6

Ingredients:

- 1lb. pork loin ribs
- 1 tsp. olive oil
- 1 tsp. minced garlic
- ¼ tsp. cumin
- ¼ tsp. chili powder

- 1 tbsp. butter
- 5 tbsp. water

Directions:

1. Mix the olive oil, minced garlic, cumin, and chili flakes in a bowl.
2. Melt the butter and add to the spice mixture.
3. Add water.
4. Rub the pork ribs with the spice mixture generously.
5. Cook the ribs for 8 hours on Low.

Nutrients per serving:

- Calories: 203
- Fat: 14g
- Carbs: 10g
- Protein: 9.8g

Easy Lamb Chops

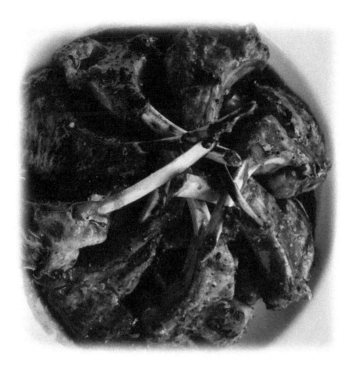

Prep time: 10 minutes

Cooking: 5 hours

Servings: 4

Ingredients:

- 4 lamb chops
- ½ tsp. salt
- 1 tsp. sesame oil
- 1/3 cup water

Directions:

1. Sprinkle the lamb chops with sesame oil, salt, and ground black pepper.
2. Place the lamb chops in the slow cooker and add water.
3. Close the lid and cook the meal on High for 5 hours.

Nutrients per serving:

- Calories: 169
- Fat: 7.4g
- Carbs: 0.3g
- Protein: 24g

Lamb With Capers

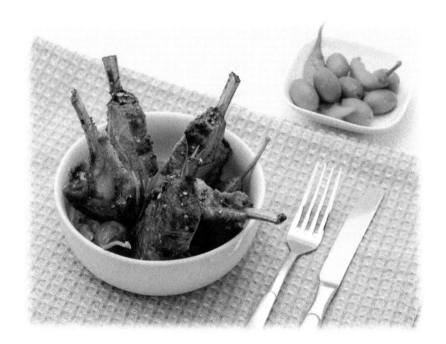

Prep time: 5 minutes
Cooking: 4 hours
Servings: 2

Ingredients:

- 1lb. lamb chops
- 1 tbsp. capers
- ½ cup beef stock
- ¼ cup tomato passata
- ½ tsp. sweet paprika
- ½ tsp. chili powder

- 2 tbsp. olive oil
- 3 scallions, chopped
- A pinch of salt and black pepper

Directions:

1. In your Slow Cooker, mix the lamb chops with the capers, stock, and the other ingredients, toss, put the lid on and cook on High for 4 hours. Divide the mix between plates and serve.

Nutrients per serving:

- Calories: 244
- Fat: 12g
- Carbs: 5g
- Protein: 16g

Lamb and Cabbage

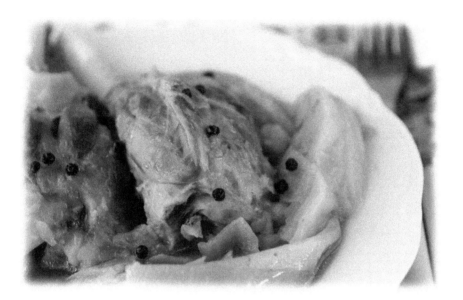

Prep time: 5 minutes

Cooking: 5 hours

Servings: 2

Ingredients:

- 2 lb. lamb stew meat, cubed
- 1 cup red cabbage, shredded
- 1 cup beef stock
- 1 tsp. avocado oil
- 1 tsp. sweet paprika
- 2 tbsp. tomato paste
- A pinch of salt and black pepper
- 1 tbsp. cilantro, chopped

Directions:

1. In your Slow Cooker, mix the lamb with the cabbage, stock, and the other ingredients, toss, put the lid on and cook on High for 5 hours. Divide everything between plates and serve.

Nutrients per serving:

- Calories: 254
- Fat: 12g
- Carbs: 6g
- Protein: 16g

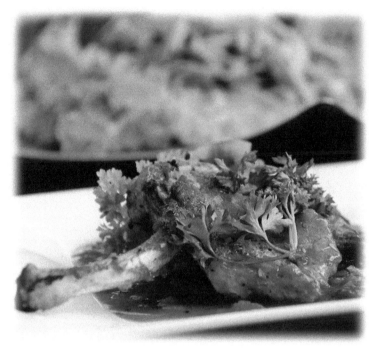

Lamb Chops with Tomato Puree

Prep time: 15 minutes

Cooking: 3 hours

Servings: 2

Ingredients:

- 10 oz. lamb chops
- 1 tbsp. tomato puree
- ½ tsp. cumin
- ½ tsp. ground coriander
- 1 tsp. garlic powder
- 1 tsp. butter

- 5 tbsp. water

Directions:

1. Mix the tomato puree, cumin, ground coriander, garlic powder, and water.
2. Brush the lamb chops with the tomato puree mixture on each side and let marinate for 20 minutes.
3. Toss the butter in the slow cooker.
4. Add the lamb chops.
5. Cook the lamb chops for 3 hours on High.

Nutrients per serving:

- Calories: 290
- Fat: 12.5g
- Carbs: 2g
- Protein: 40.3g

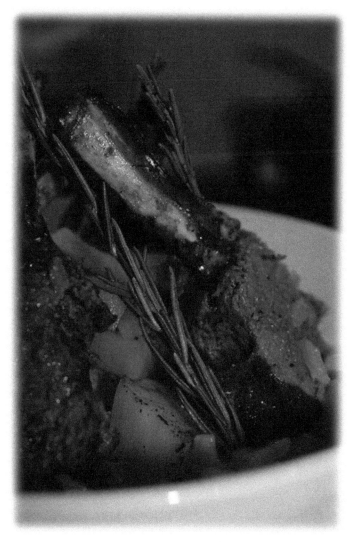

Rosemary Leg of Lamb

Prep time: 15 minutes

Cooking: 7 hours

Servings: 8

Ingredients:

- 2 lb. leg of lamb
- 1 onion
- 3 cups water
- 1 garlic clove, peeled
- 1 tbsp. mustard seeds
- 1 tsp. salt
- ½ tsp. turmeric
- 1 tsp. ground black pepper

Directions:

1. Chop the garlic clove and combine it with the mustard seeds, turmeric, black pepper, and salt.
2. Peel the onion and grate it.
3. Mix the grated onion and spice mixture.
4. Rub the leg of lamb with the grated onion mixture.
5. Put the leg of lamb in the slow cooker and cook it for 7 hours on Low.

Nutrients per serving:

- Calories: 225
- Fat: 8.7g
- Carbs: 2.2g
- Protein: 32.4g

Bay Leaf Beef

Prep time: 10 minutes

Cooking: 8 hours

Servings: 6

Ingredients:

- 1lb. corned beef
- 1 tsp. peppercorns
- 1 tsp. chili flakes
- 1 tsp. mustard seeds
- 1 bay leaf
- 1 tsp. salt
- 1 oz. bacon fat
- 4 garlic cloves
- 1 cup water
- 1 tbsp. butter

Directions:

1. Mix the peppercorns, chili flakes, mustard seeds, and salt.
2. Rub the corned beef with the spice mixture well.
3. Add the corned beef.
4. Add water, butter, and bay leaf.
5. Add the bacon fat.
6. Cook the corned beef for 8 hours on Low.

Nutrients per serving:

- Calories: 178
- Fat: 13.5g
- Carbs: 1.3g
- Protein: 12.2g

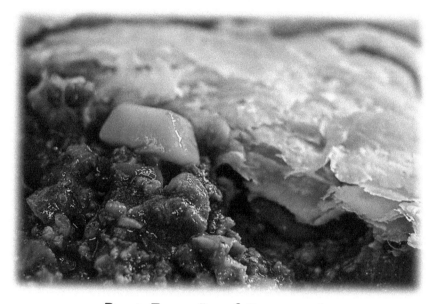

Best Easy Beef Casserole

Prep time: 5 minutes
Cooking: 6 hours
Servings: 6

Ingredients:

- 1 ½ lb. ground beef
- 1 tsp. salt
- 1 tsp. black pepper
- 1 tsp. garlic powder
- 1 tsp. paprika
- 1 cup onion, chopped
- 4 cups frozen spinach
- 2 cups white mushrooms, quartered

- 1 cup tomatoes, chopped
- 1 cup cream cheese
- 1 cup white cheddar cheese, shredded

Directions:

1. Place the ground beef in a slow cooker and season with salt, black pepper, garlic powder, and paprika.
2. Add the onion, spinach, mushrooms, and tomatoes. Stir gently.
3. Cover and cook on low for 6 hours.
4. Combine the cream cheese and white cheddar cheese.
5. Add the cheese mixture to the slow cooker and stir gently.
6. Replace the cover on the slow cooker and cook for an additional 30-40 minutes before serving.

Nutrients per serving:

- Calories: 464.6
- Fat: 35.7g
- Carbs: 13g
- Protein: 26.2g

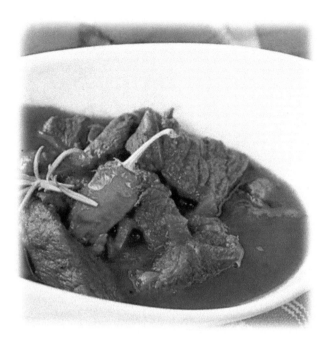

Beef in Sauce

Prep time: 10 minutes

Cooking: 9 hours

Servings: 4

Ingredients:

- 1lb. beef stew meat, chopped
- 1 tsp. garam masala
- 1 cup water
- 1 tbsp. flour
- 1 tsp. garlic powder

- 1 onion, diced

Directions:

1. Whisk flour with water until smooth and pour the liquid in the slow cooker.
2. Add gram masala and beef stew meat.
3. After this, add onion and garlic powder.
4. Close the lid and cook the meat on low for 9 hours.
5. Serve the cooked beef with thick gravy from the slow cooker.

Nutrients per serving:

- Calories: 231
- Fat 7g
- Carbs: 4.6g
- Protein: 35g

Beef With Greens

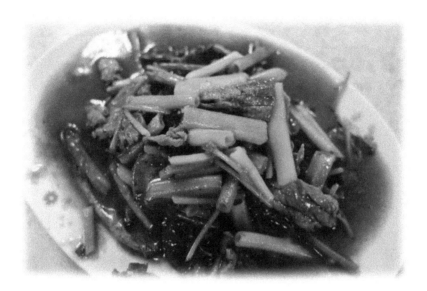

Prep time: 15 minutes
Cooking: 8 hours
Servings: 3

Ingredients:

- 1 cup fresh spinach, chopped
- 9 oz. beef stew meat, cubed
- 1 cup Swiss chard, chopped
- 2 cups water
- 1 tsp. olive oil
- 1 tsp. dried rosemary

Directions:

1. Heat olive oil in the skillet.
2. Add beef and roast it for 1 minute per side.
3. Then transfer the meat in the slow cooker.
4. Add Swiss chard, spinach, water, and rosemary.
5. Close the lid and cook the meal on Low for 8 hours.

Nutrients per serving:

- Calories: 177
- Fat: 7g
- Carbs: 1g
- Protein: 26.3g

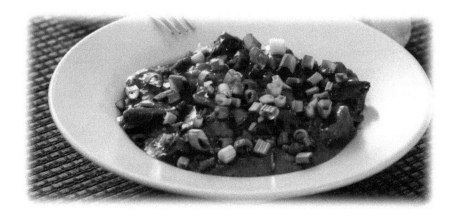

Beef and Scallions Bowl

Prep time: 10 minutes

Cooking: 5 hours

Servings: 4

Ingredients:

- 1 lb. beef stew meat, cubed
- 1 tsp. chili powder
- 2 oz. scallions, chopped
- 1 cup corn kernels, frozen
- 1 cup water
- 2 tbsp. tomato paste
- 1 tsp. minced garlic

Directions:

1. Mix water with tomato paste and pour the liquid in the slow cooker.
2. Add chili powder, beef, corn kernels, and minced garlic.
3. Close the lid and cook the meal on high for 5 hours.
4. When the meal is cooked, transfer the mixture in the bowls and top with scallions.

Nutrients per serving:

- Calories: 258
- Fat: 7.7g
- Carbs: 10.4 g
- Protein: 36.4g

Spicy Balsamic Beef

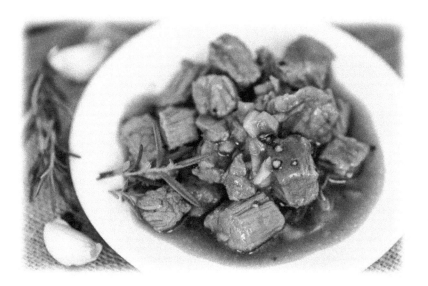

Prep time: 15 minutes

Cooking: 9 hours

Servings: 4

Ingredients:

- 1lb. beef stew meat, cubed
- 1 tsp. cayenne pepper
- 4 tbsp. balsamic vinegar
- ½ cup water
- 2 tbsp. butter

Directions:

1. Toss the butter in the skillet and melt it.

2. Then add meat and roast it for 2 minutes per side on medium heat.
3. Transfer the meat with butter in the slow cooker.
4. Add balsamic vinegar, cayenne pepper, and water.
5. Close the lid and cook the meal on Low for 9 hours.

Nutrients per serving:

- Calories: 266
- Fat: 13g
- Carbs: 0.4g
- Protein: 34.5g

Balsamic Beef

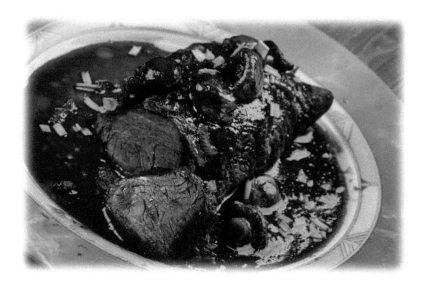

Prep time: 20 minutes

Cooking: 7 hours

Servings: 4

Ingredients:

- 2 tbsp. balsamic vinegar
- 1 tbsp. olive oil
- 1lb. beef loin
- 1 tsp. minced garlic
- ½ tsp. ground coriander
- 1 tsp. cumin
- ½ tsp. dried dill
- 2 tbsp. water

Directions:

1. Chop the beef loin roughly and place it in a large bowl, then sprinkle it with the balsamic vinegar.
2. Add olive oil, minced garlic, ground coriander, cumin, and dried dill.
3. Stir the meat well and let sit for 10 minutes.
4. Place the meat in the slow cooker and add water.
5. Cook the beef for 7 hours on Low.

Nutrients per serving:

- Calories: 241
- Fat: 13g
- Carbs: 0.6g
- Protein: 30.5g

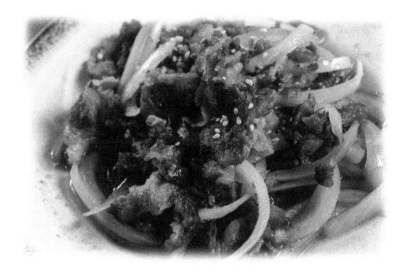

Onion Beef

Prep time: 10 minutes
Cooking: 5 hours
Servings: 14

Ingredients:

- 4lb. beef sirloin, sliced
- 2 cups white onion, chopped
- 3 cups water
- ½ cup butter
- 1 tsp. ground black pepper
- 1 tsp. salt
- 1 bay leaf

Directions:

1. Mix beef sirloin with salt and ground black pepper and transfer in the slow cooker.
2. Add butter, water, onion, and bay leaf.
3. Close the lid and cook the meat on High for 5.5 hours.

Nutrients per serving:

- Calories: 306
- Fat: 14.7g
- Carbs: 1.7g
- Protein: 39.6g

Peppered Steak

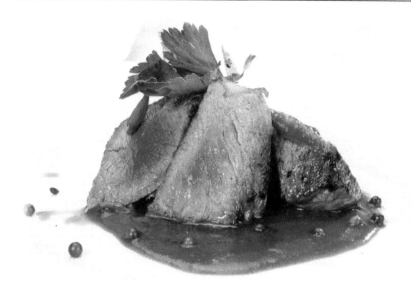

Prep time: 15 minutes

Cooking: 4 hours

Servings: 4

Ingredients:

- 10 oz. Sirloin Steak
- 3 cups water
- 1 tbsp. peppercorns
- 1 tsp. salt
- ½ tsp. ground nutmeg
- 2 garlic cloves, peeled
- 1 tsp. olive oil

Directions:

1. Make the small cuts in the sirloin and chop the garlic cloves.
2. Place the garlic cloves in the sirloin cuts.
3. Sprinkle the steak with the salt, ground nutmeg, and peppercorns.
4. Transfer the steak in the slow cooker and add water.
5. Cook the steak for 4 hours on Low.
6. Then remove the steak from the slow cooker and slice it.

Nutrients per serving:

- Calories: 192
- Fat: 12g
- Carbs: 1g
- Protein: 12g

Delightful Spicy Beef

Prep time: 5 minutes

Cooking: 10 hours

Servings: 4

Ingredients:

- 2 lb. of beef chuck on the bone
- 1 can chopped tomatoes
- 1 can chipotle sauce
- 1 can drained diced jalapeño chilies
- 1 chopped onion
- 3 cloves of minced garlic
- 2 tbsp. of chili powder
- 1 tbsp. honey
- 2 ½ tsp. kosher salt
- 1 tsp. ground cumin
- 2 cups beef broth

Directions:

1. Put all the ingredients into a slow cooker.
2. Cover and cook on low for 8 to 10 hours until the beef becomes tender.
3. Take the lid off the slow cooker during the last ½ hour to thicken the sauce.
4. Take the beef out and use a fork to shred it, and mix into the sauce in the slow cooker.

5. Divide onto plates and serve.

Nutrients per serving:

- Calories: 261
- Fat:11g
- Carbs: 5.5g
- Protein: 30g

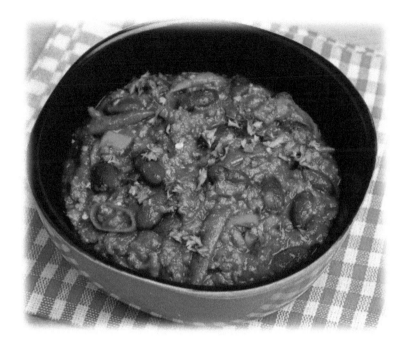

Tasty Spiced Chili Beef Eye Roast

Prep time: 5 minutes

Cooking: 8 hours

Servings: 4

Ingredients:

- 3 lb. lean ground beef eye roast
- 2 tbsp. Worcestershire sauce
- 4 tbsp. fresh lime juice
- 1 ½ cups diced onions
- 1 cup diced red bell pepper

- 3 cloves minced garlic
- 3 minced and seeded Serrano chilies
- Salt and pepper
- ½ cup beef broth
- 1 cup canned tomatoes, diced
- ½ tsp. dried oregano

Directions:

1. Use salt and pepper to season the beef and put it into the slow cooker.
2. In a large bowl, whisk the remaining ingredients together and pour them over the beef.
3. Cook on low for 8 hours.
4. Use 2 forks to shred the beef

Nutrients per serving:

- Calories: 247
- Carbs: 5.8g
- Fat: 6g
- Protein: 40g

Spectacular Meaty Crushed Tomato Bolognese

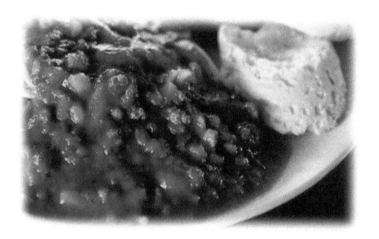

Prep time: 5 minutes

Cooking: 6 hours

Servings: 4

Ingredients:

- 4 oz. chopped pancetta
- 1 tbsp. butter
- 1 white onion, minced
- 2 stalks celery, minced
- 2 carrots, minced
- 2 lb. ground beef, 95% lean
- ¼ cup white wine
- 2 cans crushed tomatoes
- 3 bay leaves

- Salt and pepper
- ¼ cup chopped fresh parsley
- ½ cup half and half

Directions:

1. In a deep pan on low heat, sauté the pancetta for 4-5 minutes.
2. Add the carrots, onions, celery, and butter and cook for another 5 minutes.
3. Turn the heat up to medium, add the meat and the pepper and sauté until the meat browns.
4. Drain the fat, add the wine and cook for a further 3-4 minutes.
5. Pour the mixture into the slow cooker, add salt and pepper, the tomatoes, and bay leaves.
6. Cover and cook on low for 6 hours.
7. Add the half and half and the parsley.
8. Pour over pasta and serve.

Nutrients per serving:

- Calories: 143
- Fat: 7g
- Carbs: 5.4g
- Protein: 15g

Wonderful Beef & Bacon Meatballs

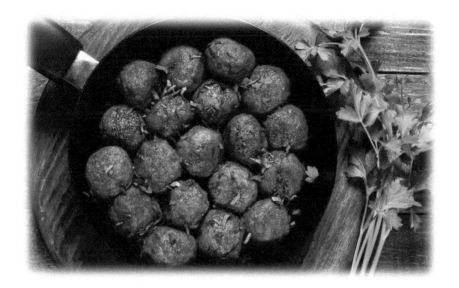

Prep time: 5 minutes

Cooking: 6 hours

Servings: 4

Ingredients:

- 2lb. ground beef
- 2 slices diced bacon
- 1 quartered onion
- 2 cloves garlic
- 1 egg
- Salt and pepper
- A handful of herbs of your choice
- 14 oz. canned chopped tomatoes

Directions:

1. Combine the garlic, onion, and bacon in a food processor and work until finely chopped.
2. Add the remaining ingredients except the tomatoes and work until the ingredients turn into a smooth paste.
3. Use your hands to mold the ingredients into meatballs and arrange them in a greased slow cooker.
4. Pour the canned tomatoes over the top, cover, and cook on high for 4-6 hours.

Nutrients per serving:

- Calorie:s 358
- Fat: 22g
- Carbs: 5.2g
- Protein: 32g

Yummy Cabbage Rolls And Corned Beef

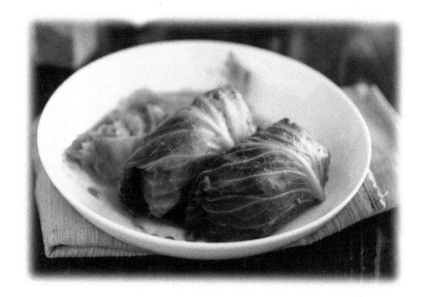

Prep time: 5 minutes

Cooking: 6 hours

Servings: 4

Ingredients:

- 2 lb. corned beef
- 1 sliced onion
- 1 lemon
- ¼ cup coffee
- ¼ cup white wine
- 1 tbsp. bacon fat
- 1 tbsp. brown mustard
- 1 tbsp. Erythritol

- 2 tsp. kosher salt
- 2 tsp. Worcestershire sauce
- 1 tsp. peppercorns
- ¼ tsp. allspice
- 1 crushed bay leaf
- 15 Savoy cabbage leaves

Directions:

1. Add the liquids, spices, and the beef to the slow cooker.
2. Cover and cook for 6 hours on low.
3. Boil a saucepan of water and add the onions and the cabbage; boil for approximately 2-3 minutes or until the cabbage leaves are soft.
4. Pour ice-cold water into a bowl and add the cabbage leaves; allow them to soak for 3-4 minutes.
5. Slice the meat and other ingredients onto the cabbage leaves and roll them tightly.
6. Squeeze the lemon over the top and serve.

Nutrients per serving:

- Calories: 478
- Fat: 25g
- Carbs: 3.8g
- Protein: 34.2g

SOUPS & STEWS

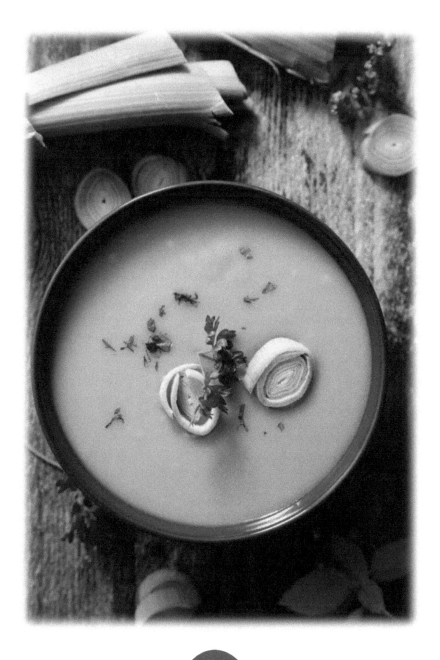

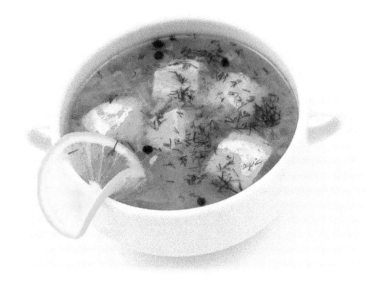

Salmon Soup

Prep time: 8 minutes

Cooking: 3 hours

Servings: 4

Ingredients:

- 2 cups water
- 1 cup coconut cream
- 1 tsp. garlic powder
- 2 garlic cloves
- 1 tsp. lemongrass
- ½ tsp. chili flakes
- 8 oz. salmon
- 1 tsp. salt

Directions:

1. Mix the water with cream and the other ingredients except the fish.
2. Cook the stock for 2 hours on High.
3. Add salmon.
4. Cook the soup for 1 hour on Low.

Nutrients per serving:

- Calories: 209
- Fat: 12g
- Carbs: 5g
- Protein 7g

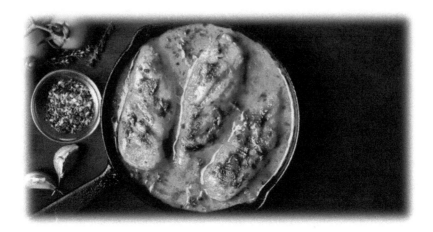

Spicy Chicken Stew

Prep time: 5 minutes

Cooking: 9 hours

Servings: 6

Ingredients:

- 3 chicken breasts, boneless and skinless
- 2 cans diced tomatoes and chilies
- ½ cup sour cream
- 1 cup onions, optional
- ½ cup Mexican cheese, shredded

Directions:

1. Place chicken breasts at the bottom of the slow cooker and top with tomatoes.
2. Cover and cook on Low for about 9 hours.
3. Dish out and serve hot.

Nutrients per serving:

- Calories: 286
- Fat: 12.7g
- Carbs: 3.8 g
- Protein: 20g

Chili Rabbit Stew

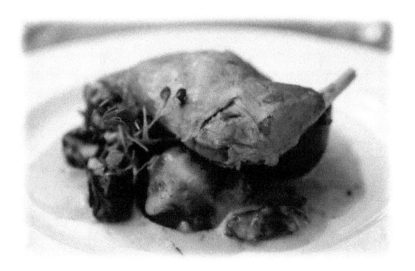

Prep time: 15 minutes

Cooking: 5 hours

Servings: 6

Ingredients:

- 10 oz. rabbit, chopped
- 2 eggplants, chopped
- 1 zucchini, chopped
- 1 onion, chopped
- 2 cups water
- 1 tbsp. butter
- 1 tsp. salt
- 1 tsp. chili flakes

Directions:

1. Place the chopped eggplants, zucchini, onion, and rabbit in the slow cooker.
2. Add water, butter, salt, and chili flakes.
3. Stir the stew.
4. Cook the stew for 5 hours on Low.

Nutrients per serving:

- Calories: 168
- Fat: 6g
- Carbs: 12.9g
- Protein: 16g

Beef Chili

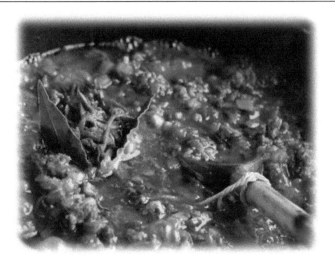

Prep time: 5 minutes

Cooking: 3 hours

Servings: 8

Ingredients:

- 2 lb. lean ground beef
- 29 oz. canned diced tomatoes, not drained
- 3 tbsp. chili powder
- 1 yellow onion, chopped
- ¼ cup tomato paste
- 1 jalapeno, minced
- 3 garlic cloves, minced
- 1 tsp. Kosher salt
- 1 tsp. ground cumin
- 1 tsp. black pepper

- 2 bay leaves

Directions:

1. Cook onions and beef over medium high heat in a pot until brown.
2. Transfer to the slow cooker along with the rest of the ingredients.
3. Cover and cook on high for about 3 hours and dish out to serve.

Nutrients per serving:

- Calories: 560
- Fat: 9g
- Carbs: 8.9g
- Protein: 30g

Broccoli Cheese Soup

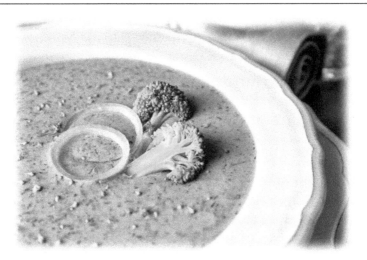

Prep time: 5 minutes

Cooking: 6 hours

Servings: 6

Ingredients:

- 1½ cups heavy cream
- 2½ cups water
- ½ cup red bell pepper, chopped
- 2 cups broccoli, chopped, thawed, and drained
- 2 tbsp. chives, chopped
- ¾ tsp. salt
- 2 tbsp. butter
- ½ tsp. dry mustard
- 8 oz. cheddar cheese, shredded
- 4 cups chicken broth

- ¼ tsp. cayenne pepper

Directions:

1. Put all the ingredients in a slow cooker except chives and cheese and mix well.
2. Cover and cook on Low for about 6 hours.
3. Sprinkle with cheese and cook on Low for about 30 minutes.
4. Garnish with chives and serve hot.

Nutrients per serving:

- Calories: 353
- Fat: 10g
- Carbs: 4g
- Protein: 30g

Cream of Sweet Potato Soup

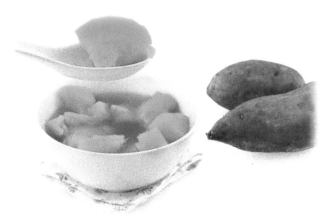

Prep time: 5 minutes

Cooking: 6 hours

Servings: 4

Ingredients:

- 24 oz. sweet potatoes, peeled and chopped
- 1 red onion, peeled and chopped
- 2 celery stalks, chopped
- 5 cups chicken stock
- 1 cup full-fat coconut milk, unsweetened

Instructions:

1. Grease a 4-quart slow-cooker and add all the ingredients to it, apart from the coconut milk.
2. Season with salt and ground black pepper, and stir to combine.

3. Cover and seal the slow-cooker with its lid, and adjust the cook timer for 6 hours.
4. Allow to cook at a low heat setting.
5. Puree the soup using a stick blender until smooth, then stir in the coconut milk.
6. Continue cooking for 30 minutes and then ladle soup into warm bowls to serve.

Nutrients per serving:

- Calories: 163
- Fat: 8.5g
- Carbs: 11.5g
- Protein: 4.6g

Taco Soup

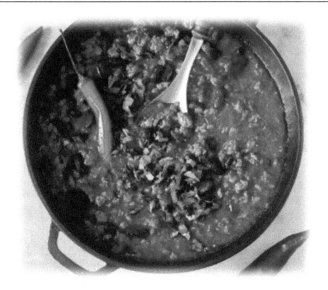

Prep time: 5 minutes

Cooking: 4 hours

Servings: 8

Ingredients:

- 1lb. ground sausage
- 2 cans chopped tomatoes
- 2 tbsp. taco seasonings
- ½ lb. cream cheese
- 4 cups chicken broth
- Fresh parsley

Instructions:

1. Place a large skillet over medium heat, pour in a tbsp. of olive oil, then add the ground sausage.
2. Allow to cook for 7 to 10 minutes, until the meat is nicely browned.
3. In the meantime, place the remaining ingredients into the slow-cooker and stir until well mixed.
4. Drain the grease from the meat and add to the slow-cooker.
5. Stir all ingredients together until well-mixed, then cover and seal the slow-cooker with its lid.
6. Adjust the cook timer for 4 hours, and allow to cook at a low heat setting.
7. Garnish with frsh parsley and cheese and serve.

Nutrients per serving:
- Calories: 547
- Fat: 20g
- Carbs: 5g
- Protein: 33g

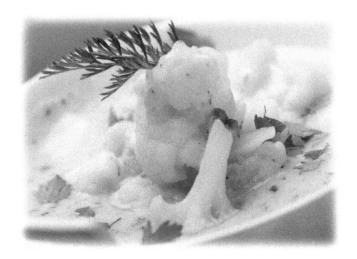

Creamy Cauliflower Soup

Prep time: 5 minutes

Cooking: 6 hours

Servings: 6

Ingredients:

- 1 cauliflower head, cut into florets
- 1 tsp. minced garlic
- 4 oz. grated cheddar cheese
- 8 oz. heavy cream
- 4 cups chicken stock

Instructions:

1. Grease a 4-quart slow-cooker and add the cauliflower florets, garlic, and stock.

2. Season with salt and ground black pepper, and stir until mixed.
3. Cover and seal slow-cooker with its lid, and adjust the cook timer for 4 to 6 hours, allowing to cook at a low heat setting.
4. Stir in the cream and the cheese, and blend until smooth using a stick blender.
5. Serve immediately.

Nutrients per serving:

- Calories: 290
- Fat: 25g
- Carbs: 6g
- Protein: 10g

Greek Lemon Chicken Soup

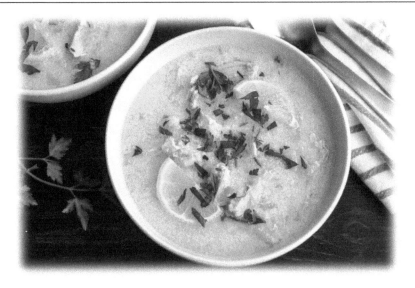

Prep time: 5 minutes

Cooking: 5 hours

Servings: 6

Ingredients:

- 4 chicken breasts, skinless
- 4 cups spaghetti squash
- 1/4 cup parsley, chopped
- 1/3 cup lemon juice, fresh
- 3 eggs
- 10 cups chicken stock

Instructions:

1. Season the chicken with salt and ground black pepper, and add to a 4-quart slow-cooker.
2. Add the spaghetti squash, parsley, and chicken stock, and stir until well-mixed.
3. Cover and seal the slow-cooker with its lid, and adjust the cook timer for 4 to 5 hours, allowing to cook at a low heat setting.
4. Remove the chicken from the soup and shred using forks.
5. Return the shredded chicken to the slow-cooker.
6. Beat the egg and the lemon juice together in a bowl, then add one cup of the hot broth mixture, stirring continuously.
7. Add this heated lemon mixture to the slow-cooker, and stir until combined.
8. Adjust the seasoning, and ladle the soup into warmed bowls to serve.

Nutrients per serving:
- Calories: 289
- Fats: 15g
- Carbs: 9g
- Protein: 33g

Tuscan Soup

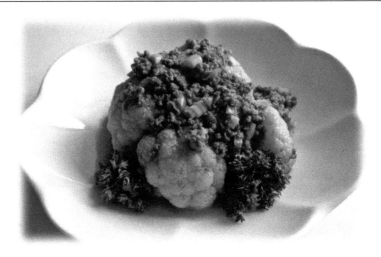

Prep time: 5 minutes

Cooking: 8 hours

Servings: 6

Ingredients:

- 6 oz. ground Italian sausage
- 8 oz. cauliflower florets
- 3 cups chopped kale
- 2 oz. chicken stock
- ½ cup heavy cream

Instructions:

1. Place a large skillet over medium heat, pour a tbsp. of olive oil onto the pan, and add the ground sausage.
2. Cook for 7 to 10 minutes, until nicely browned.

3. Drain off the fat, and transfer the meat to the slow-cooker.

4. Add the cauliflower florets, kale, and chicken stock, and season with salt, ground black pepper, and red pepper flakes.

5. Stir until mixed, then cover and seal slow-cooker with its lid.

6. Adjust the cook timer for 8 hours and allow to cook at a low heat setting.

7. Gently stir in the cream, and serve immediately.

Nutrients per serving:

- Calories: 246
- Fat: 19g
- Carbs: 3.3g
- Protein: 15g

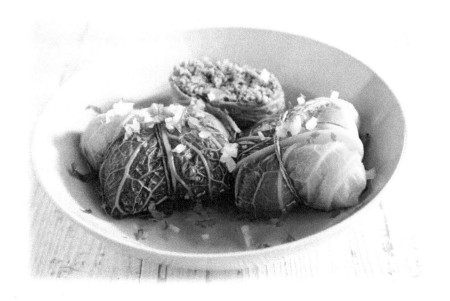

Cabbage Roll Soup

Prep time: 5 minutes

Cooking: 6 hours

Servings: 4

Ingredients:

- 1lb. ground pork, pasture-raised
- 1 cup cauliflower rice
- 4 cups sliced cabbage
- ¼ cup chopped white onion
- ¼ cup chopped shallots
- ½ tsp. minced garlic
- ½ tsp. salt

- ½ tsp. ground black pepper
- ½ tsp. dried parsley
- ¼ tsp. dried oregano
- 1tbsp. avocado oil
- 8oz. marinara sauce, sugar-free
- 3 cups beef broth

Directions:

1. Place a medium skillet pan over medium-high heat, add oil and when hot, add onion and shallots and cook for 5 minutes or until softened.
2. Add garlic, cook for 30 seconds or until fragrant, then add pork and cook for 5 to 7 minutes or until nicely browned.
3. Season with salt, black pepper, parsley, and oregano, pour in marinara sauce, and stir well.
4. Then add cauliflower rice, stir until evenly coated, and transfer the mixture into a 6-quart slow cooker.
5. Plug in the slow cooker, pour in beef broth, then add cabbage and stir until combined.
6. Shut with lid and cook for 6 hours at low heat setting or 3 hours at high setting.
7. Serve straight away.

Nutrients per serving:
- Calories: 346
- Fat: 26g
- Carbs: 6g
- Protein: 20g

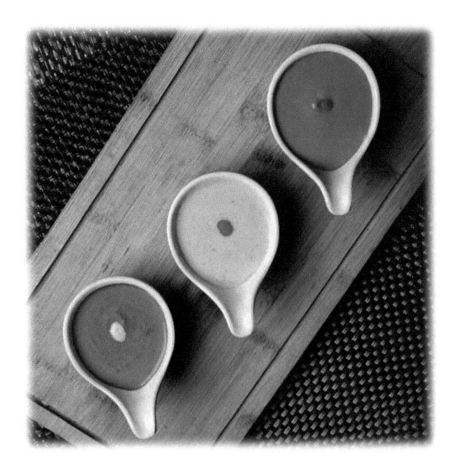

BROTHS & SAUCES

Cucumbers Pork Broth

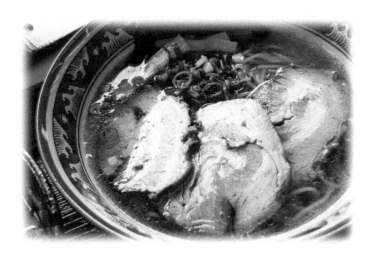

Prep time: 5 minutes

Cooking: 6 hours

Servings: 4

Ingredients:

- 1 pork butt roast, bone-in
- 1 onion, peeled and quartered
- 12 baby cucumbers
- 2 celery stalks, halved
- 4 ½ cups water

Instructions:

1. Add all ingredients to the slow cooker.
2. Cover the slow cooker and cook on low for 6 hours.

3. When the time has elapsed, strain and discard onions and celery, preserve pork and cucumbers.
4. Let rest to cool, then cover and refrigerate overnight.

Nutrients per serving:

- Calories: 119
- Fat: 4g
- Carbs: 0g
- Protein: 22g

Chicken Feet Bone Broth

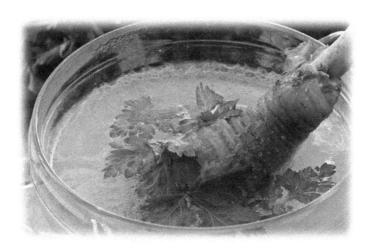

Prep time: 5 minutes

Cooking: 12 hours

Servings: 8

Ingredients:

- 12 chicken feet, pastured
- 16 cups water, filtered
- 1 tbsp. salt
- 1 sprig rosemary
- ½ inch fresh ginger

Instructions:

1. Add chicken feet, with the outer membrane removed, to the slow cooker.

2. Add water until the feet are submerged. Cover the slow cooker and bring it to a boil.
3. Use a spoon to skim off any fat on top. Add salt, rosemary, and ginger, then cook on low for 12 hours.

Nutrients per serving:

- Calories: 103
- Fat: 6g
- Carbs: 1.8g
- Protein: 10.6g

Gingery High Collagen Bone Broth

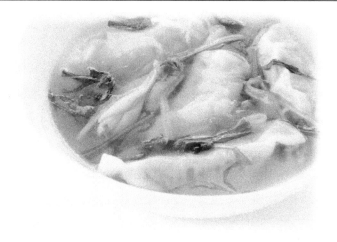

Prep time: 30 minutes

Cooking: 10 hours

Servings: 8

Ingredients:

- 2 lb. chicken wings, cut into pieces
- 1 lb. chicken feet
- 1 onion
- 1 cucumber
- 1 stalk celery
- 8 garlic cloves, minced
- 1-inch ginger, minced
- 1 tbsp. salt
- ½ tbsp. black pepper
- 4 cups water

Instructions:

1. Add all ingredients to the slow cooker. The water should submerge all the ingredients.
2. Cover and cook on high for 10 hours.

Nutrients per serving:

- Calories: 262
- Fat: 4g
- Carbs: 3g
- Protein: 22g

Vegetables and Cheese Sauce

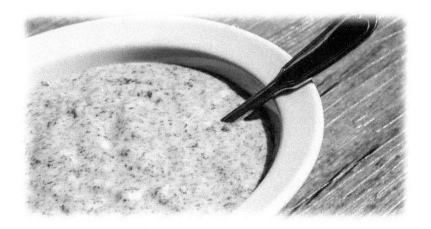

Prep time: 5 minutes

Cooking: 3 hours

Servings: 6

Ingredients:

- 16 oz. thawed Italian vegetables, frozen
- 3 cups thawed broccoli florets, frozen
- 8 oz. cream cheese, sliced
- 1 ½ cups thawed kale, frozen, cut, and squeezed dry
- ⅓ cup chicken broth
- 1 tbsp. butter
- ¼ tbsp. salt
- ¼ tbsp. pepper

Instructions:

1. Place the Italian vegetables, broccoli, cheese, kale, chicken broth, butter, salt, and pepper in a slow cooker.
2. Cover and cook for 3 hours and when all the cheese will have melted.
3. Remove the lid and stir the sauce.
4. Serve and enjoy.

Nutrients per serving:

- Calories: 240
- Fat: 17g,
- Carbs: 14g
- Protein: 10g

Beer Blue Cheese Sauce

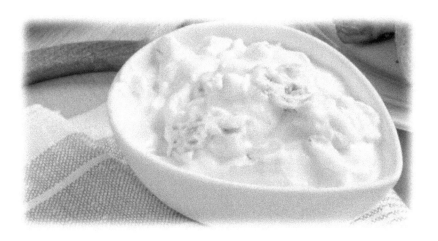

Prep time: 5 minutes

Cooking: 1 hour

Servings: 8

Ingredients:

- 8 oz. blue cheese
- 16 oz. cream cheese
- 1 cup yellow cheddar cheese, shredded
- 3 scallions, sliced and steam removed
- 1 tbsp. cayenne pepper, ground
- 12 oz. can Coors light

Instructions:

1. In a slow cooker mix, the blue cheese, cream cheese, cheddar cheese, scallions, and cayenne pepper.

2. Pour the Coors light on top of the ingredients in the slow cooker.
3. Cover and cook for 1 hour, ensuring that you stir after every 20 minutes and all cheese will have melted.

Nutrients per serving:

- Calories: 356
- Fat: 32
- Carbs: 4g
- Protein: 13g

Pizza Fondue Sauce

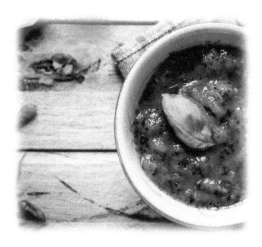

Prep time: 5 minutes

Cooking: 3 hours

Servings:

Ingredients:

- 1 lb. ground beef, lean
- 32 oz. pizza sauce
- 8 oz. mozzarella shredded cheese
- 8 oz. cheddar cheese, shredded
- 1 tbsp. oregano
- 2 tbsp. grated parmesan cheese
- Additional toppings of choice

Instructions:

1. In a skillet, brown the beef, then drain excess fat.

2. Combine pizza sauce, beef, toppings of choice, and all other remaining ingredients in your slow cooker.
3. Cook while covered for 2-3 hours on low.
4. If desired, top with dollops of ricotta cheese in the last 30 minutes of cooking; just a few drops.

Nutrients per serving:

- Calories: 328
- Fat: 39g
- Carbs: 12g
- Protein: 25.3g

Cream Gorgonzola Sauce

Prep time: 5 minutes

Cooking: 1 hour

Servings: 8

Ingredients:

- 2 cups heavy whipping cream
- 2tbsp. parmesan cheese, grated
- 4 oz. crumbled gorgonzola cheese
- ½ tbsp. Himalayan sea salt

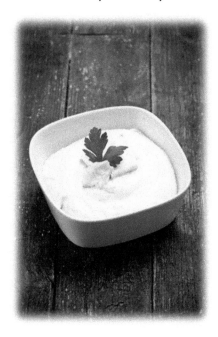

- ½ tbsp. ground black pepper.

Instruction:

1. In a slow cooker, heat the heavy cream until boiling.
2. Turn to low and let continue boiling to the desired thickness, about 40-50 minutes but don't over boil.
3. Turn off the heat, then add in all other ingredients and stir to combine.

Nutrients per serving:

- Calories: 236
- Fat: 22g
- Carbs: 3g
- Protein: 4g

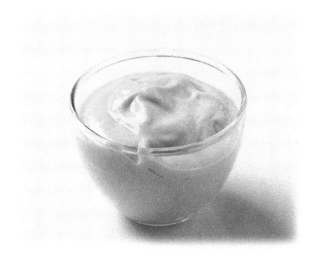

Vodka Sauce

Prep time: 15 minutes

Cooking: 6 hours

Servings: 5

Ingredients:

- Coconut oil spray
- 2 minced garlic cloves
- 1/2 chopped onion
- 1 tbsp. red pepper, crushed
- 15 oz. tomato sauce
- 1 tbsp. olive oil
- 1 cup beef broth
- 14 ½ oz. tomatoes, diced
- 5 chopped basil leaves

- 1 cup plain vodka
- ½ cup half & half
- Salt and pepper to taste

Instructions:

1. Spray the slow cooker with coconut oil spray.
2. Add garlic, onion, red pepper, tomato sauce, olive oil, beef broth, tomatoes, basil, and plain vodka to the slow cooker and mix until well combined.
3. Cover the slow cooker and cook for 6 hours.
4. Whisk in half & half to the slow cooker and cook for another 15 minutes.

Nutrients per serving:

- Calories: 316
- Fat: 11g
- Carbs: 13.9g
- Protein: 3.8g

Appendix
Measurements & Conversions

Abbreviations

Tablespoon → tbsp.

Teaspoon → tsp.

Pound → lb.

Ounce → oz.

Gallon → gal.

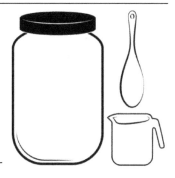

Conversions

¼ tsp. = 1 ml

½ tsp. = 2 ml

1 tsp. = 5 ml

1 tbsp. = 15 ml

¼ cup = 60 ml

½ cup = 120 ml

½ oz. = 15 g

1 cup = 235 ml

1 oz. = 30 g

2 oz. = 60 g

4 oz. = 115 g

8 oz. = 225 g

12 oz. = 340 g

16 oz. or 1 lb. = 455 g

CPSIA information can be obtained
at www.ICGtesting.com
Printed in the USA
LVHW071735290421
685992LV00025B/2380